THE LAYMAN'S GUIDE TO FOOT AND HEEL PAIN

The Layman's Guide to Foot and Heel Pain

LES BAILEY

AVENUE BOOKS

First published 2005

Published by Avenue Books
70 Milton Road, Eastbourne, East Sussex BN21 1SS, England.

ISBN 13:   978 1 905575 00 8
ISBN 10:   1 905575 00 9

Book design and production for the publisher by
Bookprint Creative Services, P.O. Box 827, BN21 3YJ, England.
Printed in Great Britain.

DEDICATED TO . . .

My beautiful wife, Sam, who manages to expertly market our clinic turning it into a major "mover and shaker", raise our lovely children, and still look a million dollars.

To the memory of Peter Bell who really started all of this.

To my sister Christine, who is firstly a wonderful sister and secondly our office superstar.

To Jill Palmer, one "heck of a journalist" who turned a small spark into a huge fire.

To Paul Williams, my colleague and brother-in-law for being a great consultant.

To Tony Robbins, Brian Tracey and all at Nightingale Conant for never-ending inspiration.

All drawings by Matt Weikop 0796 3065144.

Photography and front cover idea by Miles Winter Photography 020 8647 5805.

CONTENTS

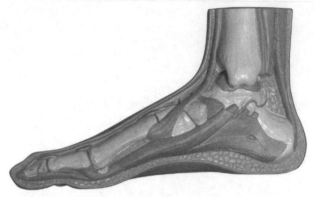

Normal foot

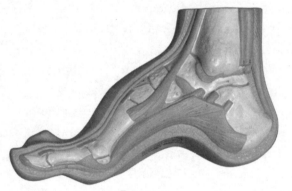

Pes cavus

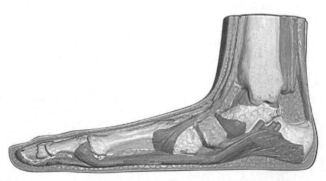

Pes planus

INTRODUCTION

I am passionate about feet! They are a miracle, an engineering marvel not even seen by the likes of Ferrari or Rolls Royce. My original training was as an osteopath, but as soon as I began dealing and specialising in biomechanics I was hooked. The way the foot works is incredible to say the least. I sincerely hope you enjoy reading this book and that in some way those beautifully designed and created vehicles on the end of your legs will benefit from you having soaked up a little knowledge from this humble volume.

"Ello, Ello, Ello!"

Many years in our distant past, there existed an ailment known to the population at large as "policeman's heel" (perhaps policeman's *hell* may have described it better) which was said to strike upon those who walk all day. Policemen used to pound on their regular beat (a rare sight nowadays) and this is where the nickname emanated from.

There were also sore feet, bad arches, and aching feet at the end of the day. One can imagine folk sat around their radiograms, feet soaking in hot water, with a glass of gin and a

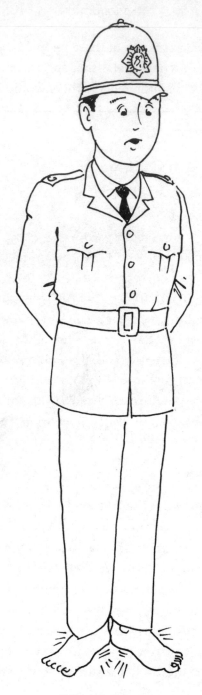

Policeman's heel

pipe full of tobacco. Some of these people who were "in the know" would purchase metal shoe inserts and just perhaps, if very lucky, gain a little relief. Others would take aspirin to

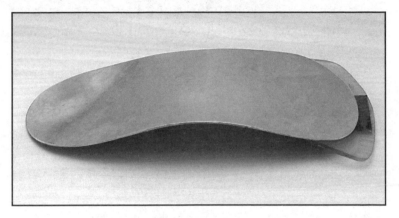

A metal shoe insert

relieve the symptoms while a great deal of the population would have consulted a physiotherapist for a dose of the latest electro-medical treatment. Ah, the bad old days . . .

But now . . .

In the 21st Century things have progressed somewhat? We have a medical name for policeman's heel which is *plantar fasciitis*, known to cause heel and arch pain in many unfortunate people. People sit round their computer games or widescreen TVs, their feet swathed in ice or rested on a hot water bottle. Some lucky people go to the local chemists and buy one of many off-the-shelf insoles, which, if very lucky, give a little pain control. Some ladies or gents opt for a visit to the doctor to be given anti-inflammatories or a locally stabbed hydrocortisone injection which generally either misses the pain site or only affords a few weeks scant relief. Many find themselves in the physiotherapist's room having a new improved electro-medical device strapped to their painful feet. Whilst others of a new age persuasion may choose chi energy crystals or organic wholemeal reflexology!

So what's new pussycat?

Excuse us for being so bold as to enquire but what on earth has actually changed? The above, past and present illustrate the fact that not a lot has actually altered over the passing of time, and symptomatic treatment is still the norm.

Whilst the medical profession have become incredibly adept at saving lives, curing diseases that were life threatening 50 years ago and bringing forth some amazingly skilled doctors and surgeons, it has done very little to effectively rid the population at large of biomechanical foot pain. Many operations have emerged for the conditions suffered by the feet, occasionally effective, but most with great risk, very little results or even the chance of more pain as a post-operative "pleasure"!

The understanding of foot pain amongst all branches of medicine is poor to say the least. GPs have very little time to understand it; most have surgeries bursting at the seams and patients with far greater and more dangerous diseases to be concerned with. A GP's life is not an easy one and with the constant stream of time wasters they encounter how would they ever get the time to specialise in foot pain? The same can be said of orthopaedic surgeons. The old and outdated operation of removing the spur has ceased. In some cases operations are carried out to release the aponeurosis, but luckily this is rare and carries with it the high risk of failure or exacerbation of pain.

The general concept of *plantar fasciitis*, in its many guises, is poorly understood by all branches of the medical profession: physiotherapists, osteopaths, chiropractors and podiatrists all seem to miss the vital point that *plantar fasciitis* is a very individual complaint, each case unique to the patient. Every case of foot pain and biomechanical misalignment has a root cause and each person is unique in their needs.

Most practitioners treat *plantar fasciitis* as a nuisance complaint rather than the painful crippling problem it really is.

Our aim is true

The aim of this book is to enlighten the lay person and hopefully stimulate further research by students and practitioners in all branches of medicine.

Even from the viewpoint of my own original training as an osteopath, a so called "complete" learning in musculoskeletal medicine, our course covered little territory into heel and foot pain. The foot as a subject was hurriedly brushed over. We seek to open the eyes of the man or woman in the street to the causes and treatments for what can only be described as a severely debilitating group of conditions.

"No-one understands!"

Do our medical practitioners have any concept of how the patient feels, with every footstep marred by dull or sharp pain? Not just one specific move, but every step? The private

practitioner who gladly takes money for short-lived temporary relief has surely never lived with the pain of those first
few steps every morning. The GP books you in to a physiotherapist who uses ultrasound and gives you stretching
exercises but all to no avail. I sometimes wonder if these practitioners have any idea of the pain felt by the patient and the
abject misery it causes.

Me? Dramatic?

Perhaps I sound a little dramatic as not all cases are absolutely excruciating. But from my side of the fence, our clinic
specialises in dealing with some of the most difficult cases of
foot pain. We see all age groups, from young children to the
very elderly, some early or mild cases and some presenting
on crutches. The one thing the longer standing cases have in
common is that they have tried every medical discipline
before arriving on our doorstep. They generally feel they
have been "through the mill" of the medical profession both
complementary and mainstream. Patients are shocked when
we locate the causative factors of their case and don't try to
fob them off with mere pain control. However, as I always
tell patients, we do have the luxury of solely specialising in
our field.

It is my belief that in order to best empathise with a condition, a practitioner should first have experienced it; so I
shall tell my own story of how I stumbled into my special-
isation.

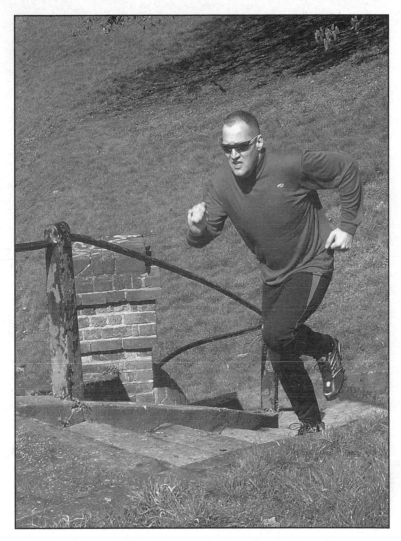

The author can now run pain free

"Run, Forrest, run!"

I was first introduced to heel pain some 18 years ago. It reared its ugly head while I was pounding the pavements on my nightly 15 mile run. Being a Thai boxing enthusiast, these runs were a necessity to maintain peak aerobic fitness and despite always running in proper running shoes, it soon became mighty obvious that the biomechanical faults in my feet were to play havoc. Not only was I experiencing heel pain, but my shin splints were getting worse by the week. To many readers, the first signs I felt will sound familiar. I thought I had trodden on a stone. My heel felt bruised and my arch felt strained and painful.

"Don't run, Forrest, don't run!"

The next few weeks saw the symptoms go from bad to worse. I employed all the usual things people try such as ice packs, anti-inflammatories, heat, massage, ultrasound; all to no avail. Eventually I saw a friend of mine who was an orthopaedic sports specialist, a doctor who spent his career in treating sporting injuries.

He treated my shin splints with hydrocortisone, a grossly painful and ridiculous procedure considering what my later research into biomechanical medicine would bring to light. He diagnosed *plantar fasciitis* with a heel spur growth which was confirmed on X-ray. This showed that the problem was not a new one and that my running, although it had forced the problem to the surface, had not been the sole causative factor. He had a podiatrist prescribe me some rigid orthotics which were made using a plaster cast. He then injected hydrocortisone into the area locally which hurt like mad. Both had very little to no effect.

My shin splints and heel pain were back with a vengeance. I was even having to use swimming as a cardiovascular exercise as I could no longer run. Even walking, whilst not as severe as I would witness in patients in later years, was a displeasure. I tried all sorts of off-the-shelf orthotics, pads, and gels from chemists and finally used some so-called orthotics from a high street foot specialist. Their staff chiropodist prescribed me some orthotic devices which caused a bruised feeling to emanate through the entire foot. They were at a complete loss as to how to adjust them and demonstrated no biomechanical knowledge whatsoever.

A very lucky meeting

It was purely by chance that I attended an osteopathic conference, something I rarely did for the reason of my poor attempts at staying awake throughout dull and uninteresting lectures. One of the trade exhibitors at the conference was a man named Peter Bell, who, little did I realise, was about to change my entire life and thrust me into a journey to the realms of biomechanical medicine. In short, Peter lead me by the nose into my specialised field. He had on display some new types of orthotics from the USA. We got talking and I told him of the problems I had personally experienced both with heel pain and shin splints. I divulged how I had tried different orthotics, which brought forth a look of amusement from Peter. After further talking I decided not to attend the next lecture and stayed with Peter for the rest of the day. He took his own particular type of cast from my feet and arranged that my orthotics would be with me in a few weeks.

For the rest of the day Peter waxed lyrical about the specialist materials used in their prescription orthotics from the USA, and how Britain is still using outdated methods of manufacture and poorly designed materials. His zest and enthusiasm got to me and, looking back, my interest in osteopathy took a downturn in favour of working with foot biomechanics.

Eureka!

Three weeks later my orthotics arrived fresh from the land of Uncle Sam and I wondered whether they really would solve my problems. On day one I inserted them and at first they felt fine. Two hours later I could have quite happily discarded them. My arches hurt like mad, but I was advised to persevere. By day two things were getting easier and by day three all pain had gone. Over the next few weeks the pain in my heels disappeared, the shin pain had abated and I was reborn back to my heavy running and training schedule pain-free. A number of minor adjustments were done to the orthotics and I was back to normal. As "easy" as that, it seemed.

Peter guided me through much post-graduate training and his own personal tuition. My life's vocation was just beginning.

I began prescribing orthotics from my clinic in Buckinghamshire where, through reputation only, I went from prescribing two or three pairs a month to being inundated with painful feet from all around the area. The conditions I was treating ranged from heel pain through to knee problems, ankle instability, sacroiliac pain and all manner of biomechanical problems. The success we had even in those early days astounded me and pleased our patients.

That was a far cry from the clinic we now have in Carshalton, Surrey, where patients come in from all over the

UK and abroad and where we prescribe the orthotics using a 3D optical foot laser linked to our specialist laboratory in the USA.

Enjoy this book and take heart. If I and thousands of others can be helped, feel sure you will.

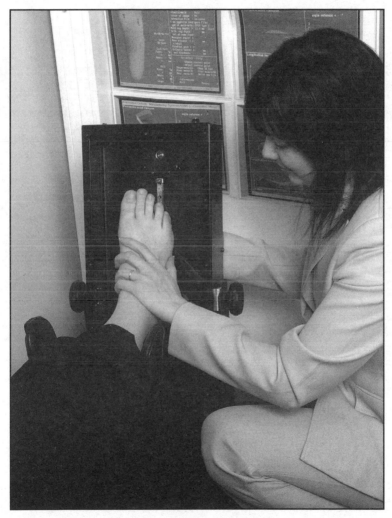

A 3D optical laser foot scanner

CHAPTER ONE

INSPIRATION FOR THE SUFFERER

We realise from many years in our field and hearing absolute horror stories from our patients that countless people go down every avenue in search of a cure for their pain, and most become very cynical. The cynicism shown is very understandable as knowledge in the field of *plantar fasciitis* is poor to say the least. However, we would like to inject a little sunshine into your life regarding the whole ghastly affair with some inspirational cases that have been treated using very specialised orthotics.

Case one: 40 years!!

Although we have treated many cases where people have suffered for ten, twenty or even thirty years, my favourite "long termer" was the prison officer who had lived with *plantar fasciitis* for 40 years. His employment necessitated him having to walk on stone floors eight hours or more every day. I cannot begin to imagine the exacerbation of pain caused by this constant pounding on hard, unforgiving concrete, day in day out. We diagnosed the case which was mainly pronation causing a constant pulling on the *plantar fascia*. Orthotics were prescribed to correct this pronation and he opted for a little manual treatment from our remedial therapist to hurry the healing along a little. Two days after receiving the orthotics he strolled into the clinic wearing a smile usually kept in reserve by showbiz personalities and . . . you've guessed it . . . pain free.

We must emphasise that not all cases go as quickly as this but, thank God, most respond rapidly.

Case 2 – A bet?

In 2002, a lady in her early thirties consulted us in quite some pain. She had been prescribed rigid orthotics made via a plaster cast from a local chiropodist. Upon examination, they had exacerbated the symptoms by literally bruising the *plantar fascia* and had thrown the feet into excessive supination by their inaccuracy. She was very satisfied with what I told her and we assessed the correct orthotics and went about laser scanning her feet. The next day her father rang me, absolutely fuming that she had spent money on what he considered was exactly what she already had. I explained why I had replaced what she had, but he was difficult to placate. After further conversation it transpired we were in the same gentlemen's club. A friendly bet was wagered that if I was wrong I would refund his daughter and buy him dinner at the club. He still owes me dinner!

Case 3 – Marathon man

Mr G. arrived at our clinic, a man in his late 40s, sporting a pair of NHS crutches, quite unable to walk unaided. He had

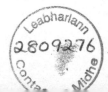

been a keen runner but had been struck down by severe *plantar fasciitis* for three years and had sported crutches for the last six months. Upon examination he presented with very high arches (*pes cavus*) and rigid, unforgiving feet. We used orthotics to "bridge" the high arch, which I will say is a procedure requiring great accuracy. The result four months later was a gentleman who was in training for our great London Marathon.

Acres of diamonds

We see our successes as acres of diamonds; thousands of happy people able to walk again pain free. I realise that when you have been in pain for a long time and had your hopes raised and dashed many times in search of a cure, it is all too easy to give up. The best advice I can give is to start from the beginning again. Wipe away mentally all you have been told about your condition and re-evaluate it. Or, as the psychologists would say, do a paradigm shift in your mind and learn to cast a new light on the challenge at hand.

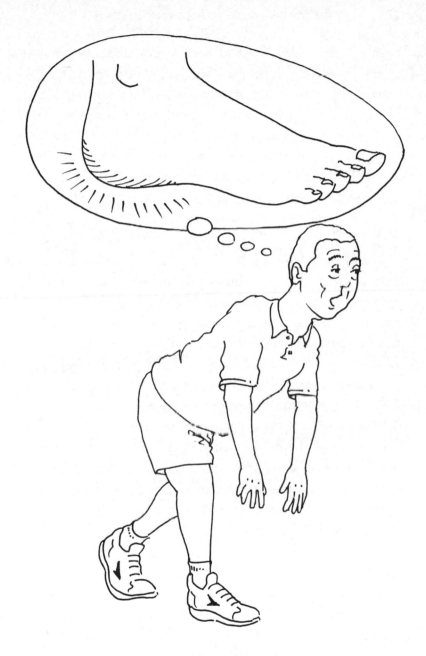

Sometimes it's all you can think of

CHAPTER TWO

THE PSYCHOLOGY OF FOOT PAIN

Those readers suffering from heel and foot pain will know only too well the abject misery of constant pain and how debilitating this can be not only physically but mentally too. The things you used to take for granted such as playing football or tennis or going on a long walk with your partner all cause pain with every step taken. Even a walk round the shops on a Saturday is a battle of wills between you and your feet, which even the best retail therapy will not cure.

The search for those magic shoes that will clear the problem goes on and on, and you live in trainers as that is what you have been told is best. You can't go out with your partner to social functions that require you to dance or stand up and what's more, your partner is beginning to feel the strain of your bad feet too.

You make vain attempts via all sorts of practitioners, but nothing works. Depression and a lack of faith in the medical profession sets in. You begin to feel low. Most practitioners tell you that it will go away soon and treat your case like a minor nuisance with as much relevance as a blackhead. To the sufferer, it is a blight on an otherwise great life.

My message is this . . . If you are a practitioner, remember, this problem is painful and debilitating. If you can't help you owe it to your patient to refer them to someone who can. With the greatest of respect, do not treat this condition like it's a minor problem – please! Should you have never experienced *plantar fasciitis* at its worst, place some marbles in your shoes at the area of the arch. Now bang the middle of the heel five or six times with a hammer. Proceed to immediately walk. After five minutes walking, remove them, walk again and, hey presto, this is a sampler of how your patient feels.

This lack of understanding extends to family, friends and colleagues. You should try to understand that they cannot see *plantar fasciitis*. The feet are in some strange social way an area of the body we never discuss. The general public's attitude toward sex, religion, race and all the old taboos may have softened almost to a point of non-existence . . . But towards feet? Ooh, not in front of the Vicar!

Now all of this is made worse by the fact that people assume because they cannot see your foot pain, that you are becoming lazy. One of the most common complaints we hear from patients is how much weight they have gained due to their painful feet. To put it bluntly, as we all know, inactivity piles on the pounds. Inactivity is also bad for the heart and circulation. Not good.

At last . . .

It is always a pleasure to see our new patients reading the reams of thank you letters we display in our waiting room. Former patients write these as a testimonial to how grateful they are. The look on the new patient's face is one of raised hope and a feeling of "at last".

In 2002, the *Daily Mirror* wrote a full page article on the work our clinic does with *plantar fasciitis*. The response was nothing short of astounding. Our phone had a maximum time of six seconds between people phoning and requesting appointments. This carried on for days, and we were kept busy for months afterwards. I mention this story here because the thing that struck me was the desperation in people's voices and the relief they expressed after. It was like they had found a drinking fountain in a desert.

Let's get positive

It has been proven time and time again that the mind, or more importantly your attitude, plays a major part in healing. Before you undertake to rid yourself of foot pain (or any disease), you must get your brain into a positive mode. Just making do with a life spent in pain is not enough. Your hopelessness and frustration leads to a depressed, angry state that leads toward giving up on ever finding a cure. The result is that no action is taken. The truth is that you have to employ massive action to get your active life back again!

Start by setting a goal in your mind and put down on paper the steps you want to take from this book to get you back to full function again. For example you may want to start with gentle exercise, hot and cold packs, a wobble board or even the ultimate step toward correct orthotics. Give your-self a timescale for each and actually write down your intentions. This will feel so powerful and positive as it puts you in charge of the journey to a cure. The mental capacity and power inside of you as a human being is so much more awesome than you could realise. Don't just sit back and accept this problem. Begin the great mental fight.

As the great sportswear manufacturers Nike said "Just do it".

No failures

When treatment after treatment fails to yield results, remember, it's not the end of the world. You or the practitioner have not failed. You have had the opportunity to ultimately discover another way that doesn't work for you. Now that has been discovered you can go on to the next method. Never give up hope. Refuse to accept any negative thoughts that you will not recover from these problems and go, go, go! You will recover and today is the first day of your new journey to a cure.

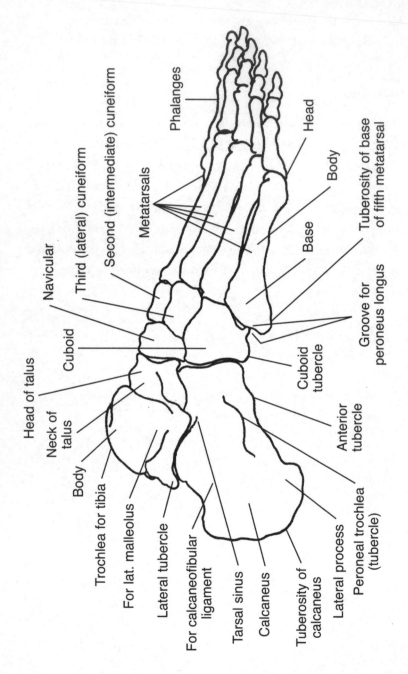

Head of talus

Neck of talus

Body

Trochlea for tibia

For lat. malleolus

Lateral tubercle

For calcaneofibular ligament

Tarsal sinus

Calcaneus

Tuberosity of calcaneus

Lateral process

Peroneal trochlea (tubercle)

Navicular

Cuboid

Third (lateral) cuneiform

Second (intermediate) cuneiform

Metatarsals

Phalanges

Head

Body

Base

Tuberosity of base of fifth metatarsal

Groove for peroneus longus

Cuboid tubercle

Anterior tubercle

Lateral view

CHAPTER THREE

RELEVANT ANATOMY

I have called this chapter relevant anatomy, as it is far from my wish to bore the lay reader with irrelevant anatomical studies that bear no relation to what they wish to learn to gain a better understanding of their own feet.

The human foot combines an amazing mechanical complexity with structural strength which is able to hold your body weight superbly. The ankle and foot serves as a foundation, shock absorber and propulsion engine. It sustains enormous pressure particularly whilst running or jumping.

It contains one quarter of the bodies bones to a total number of 26. There are 33 actual joints and over 100 muscles, tendons and ligaments. These are nourished by a huge network of blood vessels, nerves, skin and soft tissue.

This little piggy . . .

For anatomy's sake, the foot is divided into three parts; namely the forefoot (front part), midfoot (middle section) and hindfoot (the rear part). The forefoot is home to the five toes (phalanges) and their connecting long bones (metatarsals). Each toe is made up of several small bones. The big toe

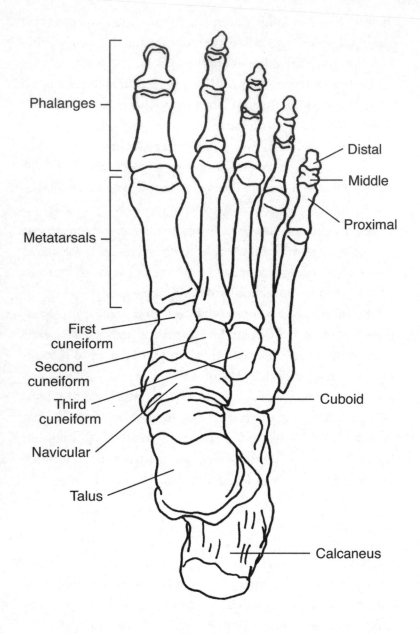

Phalanges

Metatarsals

Distal

Middle

Proximal

First
cuneiform

Second
cuneiform

Third
cuneiform

Navicular

Talus

Cuboid

Calcaneus

Dorsal view

(hallux) has two joints (interphalangeal joints) and two tiny sesamoid bones that enable it to move up and down. The other four toes have three bones and two joints. The phalanges are connected to the metatarsals by five metatarsal phalangeal joints at the ball of the foot. The forefoot bears half the body's weight and balances pressure on the ball of the foot.

The midfoot has five irregularly shaped tarsal bones which forms the foot's arch and serves as a shock absorber. The bones of the midfoot are connected to the forefoot and hindfoot by both muscles and the *plantar fascia*.

The hindfoot is composed of three joints and links the midfoot to the ankle (talus). The top of the talus is connected to the two long bones of the lower leg forming a hinge that allows the foot to move up and down. The heel bone (calcaneus) is the largest bone in the foot. It joins the talus to form the subtalar joint which enables the foot to rotate at the ankle. The bottom of this large heel bone, or "calcaneus", is cushioned from impact by a layer of fat.

A network of muscles, tendons and ligaments supports the bones and joints in the foot. There are twenty muscles in the foot that give it its shape by literally holding the bones in position and these contract and expand to impact movement. The major muscles in the foot are:-

- The anterior tibial which enables the foot to move upward.
- The posterior tibial.
- The peroneal tibial which controls movement on the outer ankle.
- The extensors which help the ankle raise the toes to initiate the act of stepping forward.

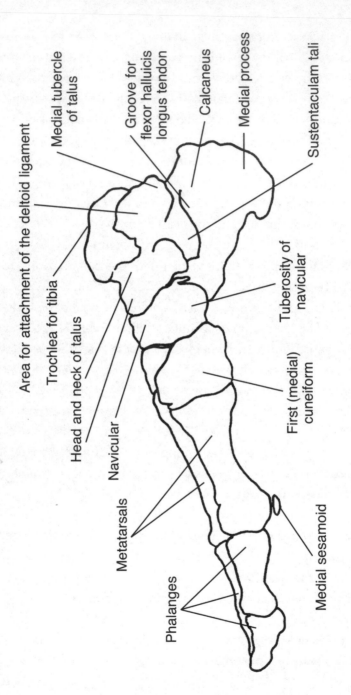

Area for attachment of the deltoid ligament

Trochlea for tibia

Medial tubercle of talus

Groove for flexor halluicis longus tendon

Calcaneus

Medial process

Sustentaculum tali

Head and neck of talus

Navicular

Tuberosity of navicular

Metatarsals

First (medial) cuneiform

Phalanges

Medial sesamoid

Medial view

● The flexors which stabilise the toes against the ground.

Smaller muscles enable the toes to lift and curl. There are elastic tendons in the foot that connect muscles to bone and joints. The largest and strongest of these is the Achilles tendon, which extends from the calf muscle to the heel. Its strength and function facilitate walking, running and jumping.

Ligaments are like the guy ropes on a circus tent and stabilise and hold everything in place. The longest of these, although not strictly speaking "ligaments", are the plantar fascia. For the best part this is our major core of interest.

What is the Plantar Fascia?

The plantar fascia and aponeurosis have a complicated and confusing "press" in many textbooks, which generally either mix everything up or over-complicate issues entirely.

The plantar fascia is composed of fibrous bands of connective tissue. It originates from the plantar medial tubercle of the calcaneum. It is made up of three distinct bands, the medial, central and lateral (1). This explains why some patients experience *plantar fasciitis* pain not only in the middle section of the arch but often in the medial aspects of the fascia, particularly in the area where the medial arch of the foot meets the heel. Occasionally, albeit in fairly rare cases, the lateral fascia experiences symptoms too.

Most textbooks are very confused as to the terms and differences in plantar fascia and plantar aponeurosis. It is also very confusing to students as to how it is made up, as some call it muscle, some refer to it as tendon and some ligament. I feel it more accurate to term it fibrous bands of connective tissue (1). The reason nature designed it like this is that muscle or tendon alone could not deal with the massively high tensile strength that runs through the fascia with every step you take.

For a more complete anatomical look at the foot and the

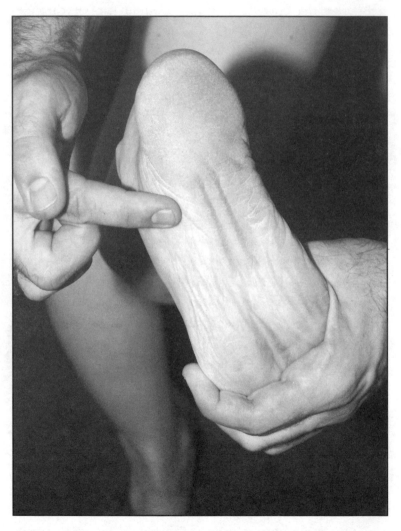

The foot flexed to expose the plantar aponeurosis

various layers of the musculature and ligamentous structures of the plantar aspect of the foot, further study would be required outside of the scope of this book. For example see references (2) and (3).

The *plantar fascia* can be considered a major tensile support network of the foot as it provides maximum support through-out the complicated gait cycle and, as I've already stated, holds up the arch of the foot during some high extremes of weight bearing. These large forces are transmitted between the hindfoot and forefoot during the stance phase of gait (4).

The plantar aponeurosis connects like a tie beam and forms the longitudinal arch of the foot. It extends from the tuber cal-canei to the ball of the foot where it attaches itself with fibres into the skin and the proximal phalanges of the toes (1).

Some sources state that the *plantar fascia* is non-elastic in that it possesses no stretch ability (5) but when diagnosing we have found different types of rigidity by palpation concurrent with different pain patterns, seriousness of symptoms and whether *pes cavus* or *pes planus*. In a nutshell, what I am saying is that not all *plantar fascia* exhibits the same rigidity (or lack of).

Other sources claim that rigidity of the *plantar fascia* comes about with age. Dr William Rossi points out, and I am in full agreement, "the ageing theory is highly debatable" (6). He goes on to state that shoeless people of advanced years rarely ever show a loss of foot elasticity. We find upon palpation no age differentiation in cases where the fibres that make up the *plantar fascia* show increased hardness or rigidity.

So we have now looked at the nuts and bolts of how the foot is constructed, in other words the basic anatomy. I hope you may be stimulated to look into this subject further and read the books and websites available. The foot is a truly

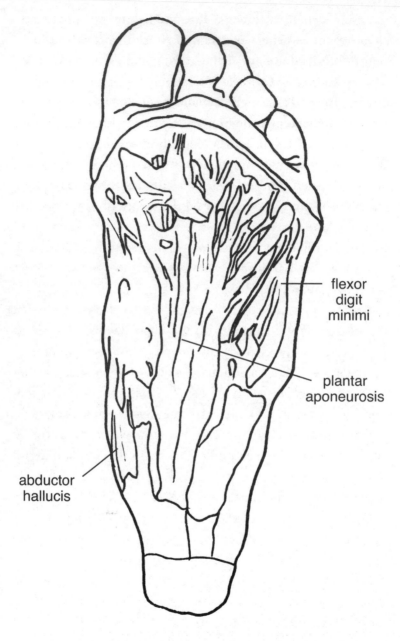

flexor
digit
minimi

plantar
aponeurosis

abductor
hallucis

Underside of foot

incredible structure and one that, even after having spent sixteen years working with them, I never tire of their many nuances and problems. For example, imagine how this amazing anatomical miracle of relatively few inches in length supports the body's weight. What is more, the feet propel the body into a walk, jog, run or sprint perfectly time after time. The feet accept their signals from the brain then set their wheels in motion, creating a beautiful synergy between nerves, muscles, tendons, bones and ligaments to carry an entire human being's weight, wherever its owner cares to take it. Truly amazing in the extreme.

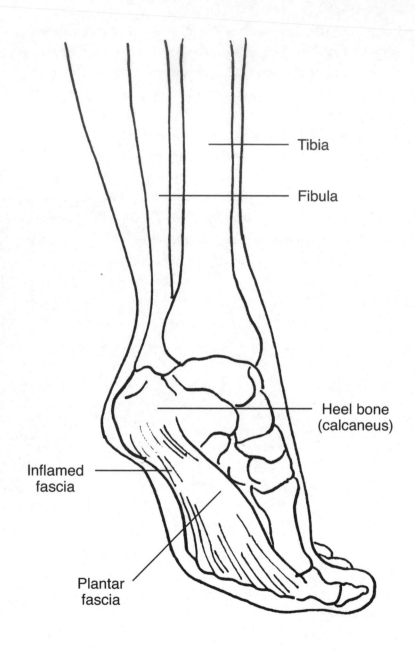

Tibia

Fibula

Heel bone
(calcaneus)

Inflamed
fascia

Plantar
fascia

CHAPTER FOUR

SO WHAT IS *PLANTAR FASCIITIS* OR "HEEL SPUR"?

Put into a simplified form, *plantar fasciitis* is a condition where the plantar aponeurosis and/or lateral and medial plantar fascia have become overstretched, perhaps a multitude of micro-tears have occurred throughout their length and possibly even slightly torn away from the heel. This tearing occurring at the calcaneum, is often called "a spur". A true heel spur very rarely causes actual pain and a high percentage of people walk around with heel spurs who have never had *plantar fasciitis* and who will never have a day's pain. An actual "heel spur" is merely a calcium growth. This has been proved to be painless, and even occurs in people who have never or will never experience pain. The sharp heel pain arises at the point of actual tear of the plantar aponeurosis at the calcaneum. This may not be torn, but can be badly inflamed. Some patients display a pain on the medial fascia at the point where the inner area of the arch meets the heel. In short, *plantar fasciitis* takes on many forms and a correct diagnosis as to your own individual cause should be sought.

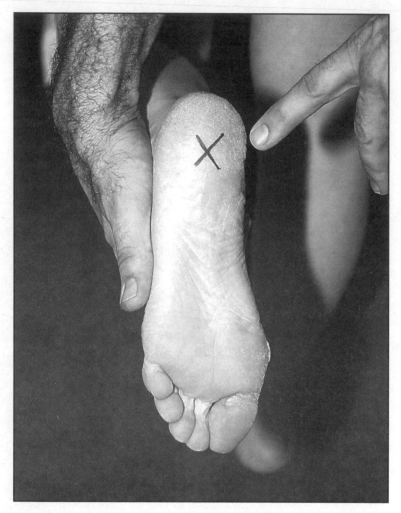

X marks the spot, heel pain site

A genetic cause?

It is modern practice in the world of psychology to blame our parents for all our physical or emotional weaknesses. From my own vast experience and observations, many of our foot problems are genetic and we gain our foot type from our parents and forefathers. Before you book yourself into counselling to discover if your parents are the root cause of your foot problems, allow me to explain my own personal findings relating to the ancestral link.

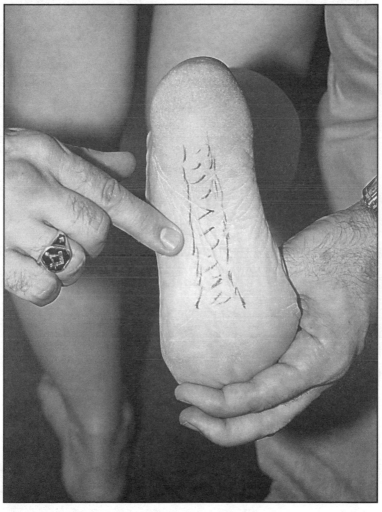

The route of the pain along the aponeurosis

I am in the fortunate position of seeing many families presenting in my consulting room; often brothers, sisters and parents. Very often a number of relatives have the same problem, but the main point to make concerning *plantar fasciitis* and its genetic connection is that although the tendency toward getting it is very often inherited, it still takes a particular activity to bring it the fore. A good example of this is that my own parents both had *plantar fasciitis* begin in their sixties which I was obviously able to clear (like my case, they are both pronators). Yet my own started in my twenties and was brought about by excessive running. The point I make is that the link to pronation and *plantar fasciitis* is very clearly a family weakness; I had "awoken" (as opposed to caused) my own *plantar fasciitis* by a heavy running schedule.

My own findings have been that around eighty per cent of people had exactly the same foot structure as their same sex parent and therefore same sex siblings. Ten per cent showed the same foot structure as their opposite sex parent and ten per cent had no similarity to either parent. Not all of the parent and sibling matches suffered the same symptoms, but very often just the same intrinsic foot structure e.g. flat feet or high arches. Very often there would be a history of the same heel problems in grandparents and patients will often tell tales of grandfather or grandmother hobbling around after rising from their bed. However, from what I have seen, the problem begins earlier in each generation. It would be wonderful if a practitioner based in a university had time to prepare official statistics on the above.

Age related

A question frequently aired by people middle-aged and over is whether *plantar fasciitis* is caused by age. The age link is of little relevance aside to comment that, in particular patients,

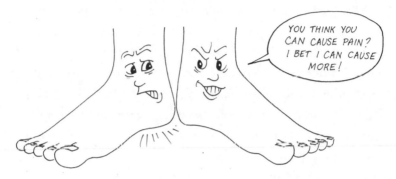

Plantar fasciitis *rarely stays in one foot before progressing on to the other*

the ligaments supporting the ankles weaken over the years causing a slow and prolonged drop to the medial arch and rearfoot, therefore exacerbating any existing pronation and placing a forceful strain on the plantar aponeurosis. This minor consideration in the age factor aside, we shall view the reasons each age group becomes prone to *plantar fasciitis*. These are not cast in stone and must be looked at as a general overview.

Childhood cases

It is often assumed that all childhood heel or foot pain is brought about by severs disease which we shall cover in a later part of the book. A big surprise to many practitioners is that children, as well as adults, do get *plantar fasciitis*. It would appear obvious that deterioration to the elasticity of the plantar aponeurosis is not a cause at this age. Our diagnostic eye will immediately turn toward a faulty biomechanical foot posture such as excessive pronation or cavus. One finds the child is generally of the hypermobile body type; in other words all the ligaments of the body "overstretch" and in the case of the feet, a pronation occurs due to this. A rarer cause we occasionally see is where the child has been born with a rigid and unmalleable plantar aponeurosis that will allow no elastic movement during the gait cycle and merely presents with a series of micro tearing along the aponeurosis length. We see this type in people of all ages, but this will tend toward presenting itself in children where the child is particularly active, for example in weight-bearing sports.

The art of prescribing orthotics to children is not to over-correct the foot to the point where it cannot strengthen during growth. As prescribers we seek to correct to the point of relieving pressure from the aponeurosis by either "bridging" a rigid aponeurosis or cavus foot or by supporting a pronator or "flat foot". I hope this reinforces my point about not using inaccurate arch lifts (even as only one example of this!). At the risk of repeating my text, we correct only to this point and not to the full correction that we would seek to achieve in most adult cases.

As a footnote, I will add that having observed many childhood cases to whom I have given repeat prescriptions over the years, I can say that "once a pronator, always a pronator". Things do not generally improve and orthotics will be a desirable prophylactic against pronatory pattern foot and limb problems for life.

Teenage/early 20s

In general terms there is often a history of partaking in competitive sports, or where a tough training regime has been followed, perhaps even into the early 20s. Before the reader accuses me of blaming the activity for the *plantar fasciitis*, may I plead a definite "not guilty". If sporting activity (or any other weight-bearing activity for that matter) had caused the problem, then all sports people would suffer from *plantar fasciitis*. The message I am trying to get across and one that I instil into our patients is that *plantar fasciitis* and other foot problems happen because you are biomechanically prone to get them. It's as if you are programmed (like a computer) from birth, that one day, out of the blue, one of these problems will occur. All it takes is for you to carry out an activity that will "awaken the sleeping beast". So in effect, the activity is merely an irritating factor and not a directly causative one. Does this make sense? If not, with all the greatest respect to the reader, please read the passage again. It is a most important factor in all ages, but is particularly poignant in young, sports people. I make no apologies for repeating the above point throughout the book, albeit in different ways, because it is a most vital part in the understanding of the "whys" of *plantar fasciitis* and the plethora of biomechanical foot ailments.

Some cases of *plantar fasciitis* in this age group will present simply because they are so pronated, or biomechanically unsound, that the plantar fascia and/or aponeurosis is under so much stress that the usual problem occurs with tearing and inflammation throughout.

Middle aged or elderly cases

It is unusual to encounter a *pes cavus* foot presented by a middle aged patient with heel pain. Not unheard of, but unusual. Generally speaking the *pes cavus* subject has had

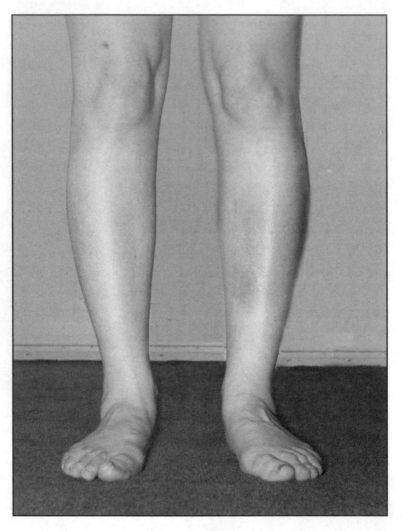

Pronation

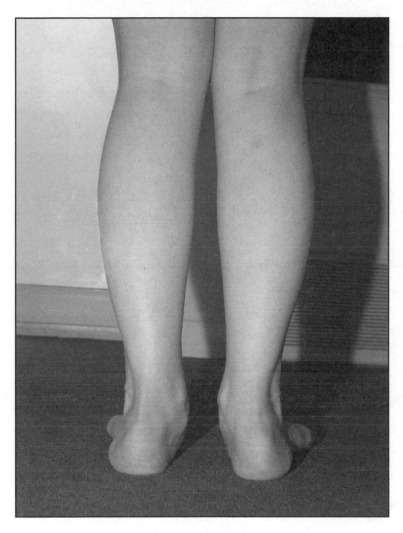

Pronation rear view noting "bowed" Achilles

plantar fasciitis at a much earlier stage in life. The exception to this is that at this age the ligaments, tendons and connective tissues become more brittle and likely to tear – the plantar aponeurosis being no exception to this – and is liable to a sudden outbreak of tearing and inflammation at this time of life. This is particularly so with *pes cavus* cases with their naturally rigid plantar fascia.

The older patients we see tend to fall into a number of causative factors. Firstly it must be understood that there must be an underlying biomechanical reason for the prob-

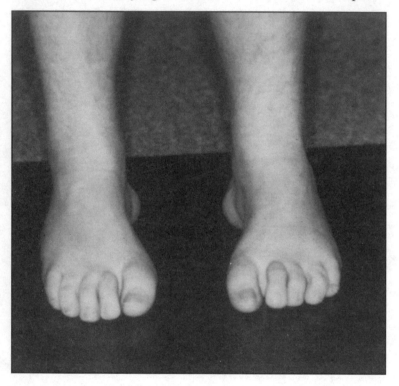

Pes cavus

lem. For example, the person will have always been pronated either midfoot, rearfoot or both or, as we have already stated, a *pes cavus* foot shape may be the root of the trouble. In the case of the pronator, it generally transpires that the pronation is worsening and causing new and more tenacious "pulling" effects on the plantar aponeurosis. This further pronation happens because the ligaments holding the foot and ankle stable weaken naturally as we age. Having stated this we must resist the temptation to assume *plantar fasciitis* or any other foot problem is merely down to age as an actual causative factor. With your new knowledge of actual tangible root causes I hope the above makes sense. Age may more accurately be thought of as an irritating factor rather than causative.

An interesting consideration . . . Asian foot

In our clinic we receive a high number of Asian patients mainly of Indian origin. I will be honest and say that I have never read or even heard of Asians showing a higher propensity to acquire *plantar fasciitis* but I shall share with the reader my own unique observations on this matter. I shall not be so arrogant as to claim that this is 100 per cent unique, but I repeat that I have never heard of this being observed before. If any professional readers care to write and correct me I shall happily consider their findings. I am certain that many practitioners of physical medicine have noticed that their Asian patients show a marked propensity toward hypermobility to the musculoskeletal structures. I certainly noticed this in my former work in osteopathy when I treated the entire human framework.

When we look at India through the eyes of an observer of yogic principles, we see it is taught and practised with great relish and its Indian participants can bend into wonderful positions easier than their Western counterparts. From this, we begin to see how this hypermobility is a reality. When we observe the anatomical make-up of the plantar aponeurosis and its similarity to a ligament, or we look at the actual ligaments of the foot and ankle, we see how the hypermobility factor irritates the tension of the plantar aponeurosis. I have further observed a phenomenon within my Asian patients and that is they seem to suffer more pain than do other nationalities suffering the same condition. The only conclusion I can reach on this matter is that the ligamentous hypermobility in the ankles must be playing its part by creating a greater tension in the aponeurosis, and therefore the heel, than in Western patients. One of my Asian patients made a very poignant remark when I told him of my findings and theories concerning Asian foot. He pointed out that many Asians in the UK, including himself, own shops which necessitates them having to stand for long periods on hard floors. Naturally this is an important consideration, but only to the effect that this lifestyle can worsen an already existing propensity to the problem. In other words, standing on hard floors does not act as a causative factor but merely as an aggravating one.

CHAPTER FIVE

A LOOK AT EVERYDAY BIOMECHANICS

Our feet are a far cry from being static structures and correct movement is absolutely essential to the health of the structures of the foot, as well as to the musculoskeletal structures above the foot such as the knees, hips and lower back, even as far as to the temporomandibular joint (jaw), according to some sources. It is the combined and interrelated function of the bones, ligaments, muscles and joints that drives the amazing engineering feat we call our feet, to propel the body and enable them to cope with the various walking surfaces we force them to tackle. One of the most complex and poorly understood roles of our feet is in their intrinsically brilliant role of shock absorption.

Any degree of loss of the foot's ability to absorb shock, or a poor or ineffectual imbalance of shock absorption will lead to faulty weight distribution. This is at the very heart and soul of nearly every foot problem. This is also at the very helm of why drug therapy is rarely ever the answer and the judicious use of intelligently designed orthotics must surely be our golden goose.

One of the shock absorbing factors as well as the natural springiness of the foot's structure, is the heel pad. This layer must play its part by padding the foot strike at its final meeting with the ground.

We very occasionally use a computerised foot pressure pad at the clinic as one aspect of our diagnostic work. This computerised pad shows where excessive pressure is landing upon standing. We generally observe that when a *plantar fasciitis* case stands on the pressure mat, it is on the heels that the main pressure shows. We rarely use this machine as our clinical experience is beyond this; but it is of interest if only to show

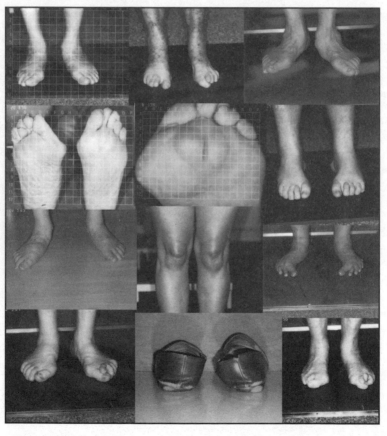

Varied problems!

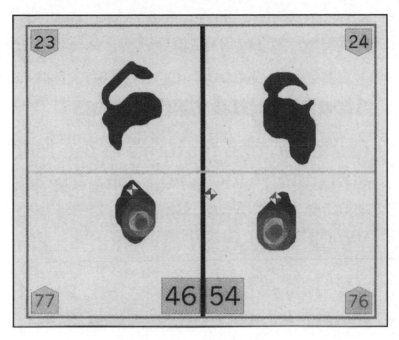

A pressure pad reading

biomechanical imbalance in picture form. The completion of the shock absorbing effect is in the eccentric contractions of the foot muscles. Imagine, if you will, the suspension in your car and how this moves each wheel up and down upon uneven surfaces. This is the effect of the eccentric contractions.

The absolutely remarkable work of the foot may be amply illustrated by its innate ability to cope with not only flat surfaces, but irregular areas such as the unforgiving "underfoot punishment" of a stony beach, cobble-stoned street or dried bumpy grassland. The foot does this frankly applaudable work by sharing the load between the forefoot, hindfoot, arch and ankle to move, like Byron's poetry, through a sea of natural and counter-balanced motion. The healthy foot glides through these motions neither landing heavily or unevenly, nor firing shockwaves throughout the body.

It is absolutely vital that the foot can cope well with uneven surfaces by showing enough flexibility to, say circumnavigate a stone yet remain rigid enough to push-off and propel the body without collapsing at the ankle.

Furthermore, in relation to our friend the plantar aponeurosis, the foot has to display a relaxed form upon standing still, yet be able, without pain, to contract adequately to assist in propelling the body to walk. This fine and dandy balance can only be achieved by a biomechanically healthy foot.

The types of foot affected

There is no one single cause of any type of foot malady, but I would like to simply explain the problems associated with the different types of foot affected. The following is obviously

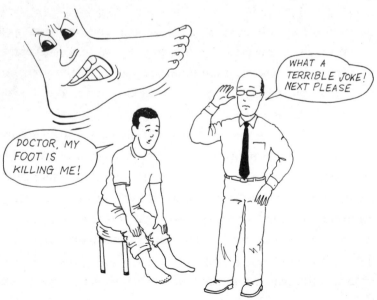

a simplified view and many other diagnostic factors must be added to the equation to extract exact causes and effect a solution.

The most challenging and my personal aesthetic favourite, is the *pes cavus* foot. This is the proud-looking foot, standing tall and rigid like a stag about to do battle. Its high arch and sloping dorsum surface (upperfoot) give it a sleek appeal resembling the shape of a stiletto shoe. But this is where the svelte and parallel beauty ends. The high arch makes this an unforgiving beast, rigid like an oak tree in a high wind, liable to break. Its plantar fascia is like tight, brittle wire, rigid and fibrous. This, coupled with the fact its other structures and supports follow suit, is equally unforgiving. This means that the plantar aponeurosis is shorter than usual and almost inevitably acquires either *plantar fasciitis* or metatarsal pain, if not only because all the person's weight is exacted upon the heel and metatarsals, whilst the arch is pulled taut like Robin Hood's bow-string pulling at the insertion in the heel and its joinings at the metatarsal heads. This makes the heel and metatarsal heads behave like two opposing tug o' war teams, ripping at the aponeurosis like weight on a rotten rope.

The pronator or flat foot is the second type in line for discussion. In this case the inner ankle slumps further inward as if trying desperately to meet up with its opposite ankle. Or, one may view it as if it were weak through alcohol and unable to bear its own weight; the arches fall flat like deflated balloons. Pronation brings with it many "veritable delights" from the multitude of musculoskeletal shortcomings including ankle pain, shin splints, knee symptoms and certain lower back imbalances.

The major negative issue in the case of *pes planus*, or flat feet, is not only in the resultant stretching of the plantar fascia (medial and aponeurosis) but also the heel strike which forces the unfortunate owner of *pes planus* feet to thump across the floor with a thud like a migraine. This has the effect of striking the heels with each step thereby exacerbating the overall problem somewhat. Therefore, when prescribing an orthotic, I always design its effect to absorb heel strike in these cases.

The pronator, like the *pes cavus*, is placing constant strain on the plantar aponeurosis and fascia by exerting a pull-like effect throughout the entire length. This pulling is caused by the collapsing effect of both ankles and arches pulling the aponeurosis away from the heel and pulling at the metatarsal heads. The result of this is micro-tearing and inflammation along the fibres.

CHAPTER SIX

THE SHORTCOMINGS OF "STANDARD" TREATMENTS IN THE UK AND EUROPE

We sit in our consulting rooms every day at our clinic and hear our patients reel-off long lists of treatments they have tried for their biomechanical foot ailments, be these plantar fasciitis or any of the plethora of conditions. These treatments are meted out by practitioners with little experience in this

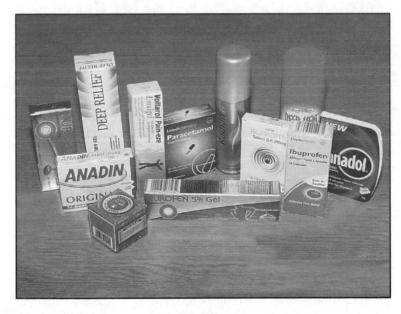

Painkillers

field, or grabbed off the shelf of a pharmacy or high street so-called foot specialist.

My first therapeutic "swipe" shall be at the vast majority doled out by practitioners. These include the rock-hard plastic type favoured by podiatrists and the "cut round your foot and hope for the best" ones found within the NHS and orthopaedic shoe makers everywhere. This is not forgetting the absolute myriad of orthotics and insoles available from chemists and shoe or sports shops. The problems encountered with these is the sheer lack of accuracy both in shape and flexibility of body; in other words the orthotics' ability to cope with individual foot rigidity or patient weight. For further views on orthotic type and structure please see my later chapter on orthotics.

Hydrocortisone is a common choice amongst doctors and orthopaedic specialists and is given out with alarming regularity. It would appear to be issued in much the same way as painkillers. My own stance on this is that cortisone can only hide chronic *plantar fasciitis* for a short time. Whilst cortisone is useful in many musculoskeletal injuries of a more acute nature, its sole use as a treatment modality for *plantar fasciitis* is short-sighted and really offers little or no benefit. My reasoning for this is that one cannot hope to fire anti-inflammatory drugs directly into the torn area and cure the condition. Surely our biomechanical eye must look toward stopping the tearing in the first place and weeding out the problem at source instead of merely cutting the flower from the weed. It has been shown time and again that overuse of hydrocortisone weakens the very tissue it is aimed at treating. One would rationally assume that we would seek to strengthen the plantar aponeurosis and not weaken it further. Jumping off my soapbox for a moment, the prudent use of cortisone can be useful in cases where the correct orthotics are used, but eventual healing is slow and stubborn. I occasionally recommend its use in some rare cases; but this is not routine, and other palliative methods should be tried first.

In my opinion, night splints and stretching exercises both fall into the same category as far as *plantar fasciitis* is con-

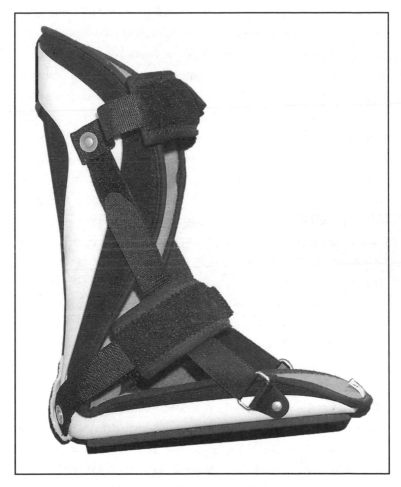

A night splint

cerned. These stretching exercises are handed out in phys-
iotherapy rooms and doctors' surgeries, osteopaths' and
chiropractic clinics up and down the UK. Let's get one thing
clear. Stop doing these now. What must be borne in mind is
that *plantar fasciitis* is a tearing and inflammation along the
shaft of the aponeurosis or even at the actual heel insertion.
View this in your head and imagine what a stretching exercise will do to a structure already torn. It worsens the tear!
What this means to the patient is that these stretches are literally opening the tears further and risking making them
worse. The so-called night splint, which looks for all intents
and purposes like a torture boot, holds the foot in a position
known as dorsiflexed which holds the tearing open
throughout the sleeping hours which is when these are
worn. Night splints mean that when the patient first stands
in the morning they do not get that dreaded searing pain
throughout the heel and arch. We see this as a negative
effect as it is not allowing any healing of the tears. The
reason the subject suffers this when not wearing night
splints is that upon standing, the patient has re-opened the
tiny tears at the heel or along the aponeurosis shaft from
where they have undergone the first stage of healing whilst
being non-weight-bearing during sleep. Therefore night
splints are aimed at literally holding these tears open so that
the foot does not initiate that first stage of healing.

Anti-inflammatories are generally the first port of call by
the family doctor. As anyone knows, pain killers and anti-
inflammatories are used to hide pain and do not have any
positive effect on the healing process of any foot pain. Aside
from this, certain of these can exhibit unpleasant side effects
such as digestive problems etc. We often see patients given

local anti-inflammatory gels. I fail to see how these can hope to penetrate the thick layer of skin on the plantar surface of the foot. I can honestly say I have never spoken to a patient who has found these gels of any use whatsoever in this area of the body.

The work of the manual therapist such as the physiotherapist, osteopath or chiropractor can play an important part in the overall picture of healing where foot problems are concerned. They may employ laser, ultrasound, deep tissue massage, interferential or even manipulation to encourage the area to heal. However, like cortisone, all this great work will be a waste until the foot is returned to its absolute correct biomechanical position and function and we have therefore tackled the cause.

Operations are a topic patients often discuss with us and they seek to find out our opinion on whether an operation

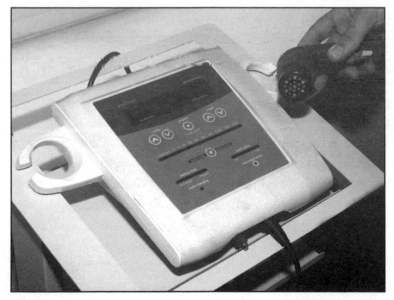

Laser machine

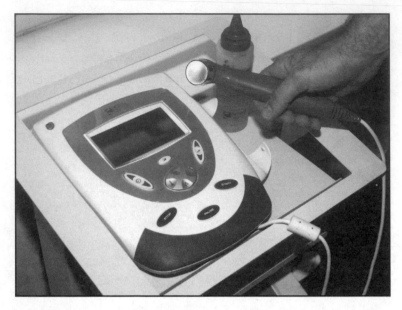

Ultrasound

will end their *plantar fasciitis*. Firstly the surgical excision of the so-called heel spur is a method that has thankfully fallen out of favour. It was a pointless exercise as the spur is actually a shelf, which it has been proven causes no pain whatsoever. The pain arises from the tearing at the heel insertion of the aponeurosis and not the spur. Other surgical methods aim at releasing the plantar fascia's tightness by making multiple stabs along its shaft or peeling off the first layer of fascia. I am none too keen on these methods except in very extreme circumstances: and I mean exceptionally rarely! I have borne witness to cases where these operations have been done and at best they have been ineffective and at worst exacerbated the problem. The cases we see post-operatively are still in need of orthotics as the cause itself has not been tackled. I will not delve too deeply into the procedures used in the operating theatre; but for those readers of a medical persuasion I heartily recommend a book called *Disorders of the heel, rearfoot and ankle* by Ranawat and Positano (see note (1)). This is a medical volume for medical people, but it is my personal favourite for further reading and study.

CHAPTER SEVEN

SELF-HELP FOR HEEL AND ARCH PAIN

Self-help is a wide ranging and very subjective topic and con-jures up images of old ladies mixing up herbal lotions and potions. You may single-out or use a mixture of some of the ideas in this chapter. They are not meant as a substitute for professional help as a full and accurate diagnosis should first be sought.

Much of the information here can be extremely useful to assist in alleviating a certain amount of the pain, and patience and perseverance will be the key.

Hot and cold packs

One of the most powerful anti-inflammatory methods is the hot and cold pack. It rapidly reduces inflammation by pumping fresh blood into the area (hot) and then dissipating it (cold). This literally opens and closes the blood vessels "squeezing" the inflammation away.

For the application of cold I recommend an ice pack or a number of these. So you will need to keep them lined up in the freezer and constantly cold. These can easily be obtained from a chemist or sports shop.

To give you your heat source one may choose a wheat pack that is heated in a microwave, a hot-water bottle or even an infra-red lamp. To be perfectly frank heat is heat, whatever the source.

The correct method of application is to place the hot pack on for five minutes, followed immediately by the cold pack and repeat as often as you wish or have time for. Try this first for perhaps four times of each as I wholly recommend a 'tester' to ensure you are not one of those rare people who react adversely to this.

I would like to share with my readers an example of how powerful hot and cold packing can be. I remember a case from when I practised as an osteopath which illustrates the remarkable effects that can be achieved employing this method. A patient consulted me, with his wife in tow. The gentleman was in a terrible state displaying a massive crisis to the sacro iliac joint. They were at great pains to point out that a major financial loss would occur if he were not out of pain in twenty-four hours or at the very least active enough to carry out the work he had been assigned.

There was severe inflammation and misalignment to the sacro iliac joints which I immediately corrected with osteo-pathic manipulation, and dissipated the cause. However this still left a great deal of inflammation which could have taken days to clear. I told them of the hot and cold treatment and realising how desperate they were, explained carefully that if they carried out hot and cold treatment for eight to ten hours continuously he should be back on his feet the next day. The credit goes to this man's wonderful wife who painstakingly did a ten-hour shift of constant hot and cold. To rid the area of that much inflammation in that short a timescale took a miracle. Hot and cold and perseverance provided that miracle.

Shoe padding

In the absence of a proper orthotic you may find shoe padding a useful temporary relief. Please bear in mind the negative effects an off-the-shelf orthotic can have, and do not

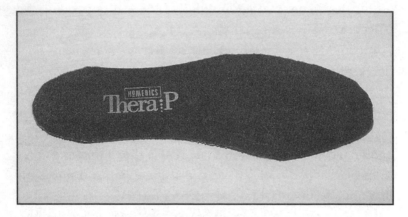

Shoe pad

use any device that is shaped. That is to say avoid, for example, those that have a shaped arch. It is preferable to use a flat bed of sorbothane that can be obtained from a sports shop, or a material with a similar shock-absorbing nature. This can act as a useful temporary "padding" and alleviate a little of the pain from the shock of walking.

Stretching

I am very cautious regarding stretching, as with *plantar fasciitis* we have areas of the foot actually torn, albeit micro tears, and we do not wish to exacerbate this by over-stretching. I rarely, if ever, recommend our patients to do stretching exercises once they have orthotics as these simply will not be needed.

A useful stretch that can be done if your case is not too

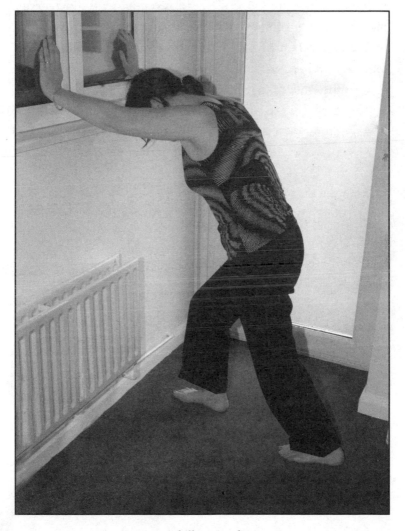

Achilles stretch

severe is the Achilles/aponeurosis stretch. This is a fairly common exercise given-out by manual therapists. I prefer the stretch to be done only after thoroughly warming the Achilles tendon and aponeurosis with either a hot water bottle, a bowl of hot water or a heat lamp. This has the effect of drawing more blood to the area and making the two areas more malleable and so less likely to tear further.

The method for this is to heat the areas thoroughly for ten minutes. When warmed throughout place both hands against the wall, place the unaffected leg in front for support and keeping the back (affected) foot flat on the floor, bend the knees and feel the Achilles and aponeurosis stretching. Do not over-stretch and immediately stop if this causes pain. Done correctly and with caution this will have the effect of making the area feel more flexible. Obviously how you react to this depends on individual factors, but on the whole it should prove a positive exercise.

Strapping

The aim of skilled strapping is the same as for orthotics. Its purpose is to bind the foot so that the arch is lifted and all strain is taken from the plantar fascias. It is not as distinctly accurate as orthotics and suffers the drawback that it would have to be redone every time you wanted to shower. However, done properly it is still my favourite temporary fix, if a little fiddly. A sports-trained physiotherapist or osteopath could possibly teach you how to carry this out at home.

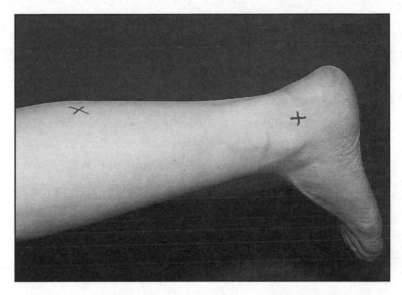

Acupressure points B1 57 and 60

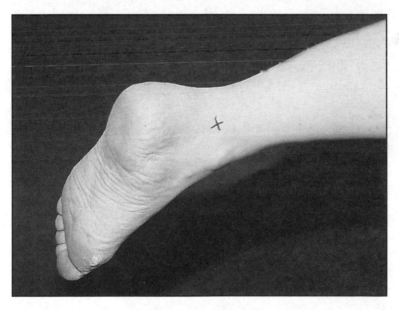

Acupressure point K3

Acupressure

Some people find acupuncture helpful for pain control and you may wish to visit an acupuncturist for this, or try acupressure to acupuncture points at home either using fingertips or a tens machine. Do not over stimulate the points but "coax" them with firm pressure.

The photographs illustrate the points (7) but one may also use "Ah Shi" or local points of tenderness (that is areas directly around or over the pain area that are particularly tender). Stimulate these by fingertips for three to five minutes at each point. You should find that this will have the effect of taking the edge off the pain.

Rest

Obviously long term rest will help with pain; but this is no long term answer, as we do not desire to live our lives in bed or on the couch. Many doctors cite rest as a major healer of foot pain; unfortunately they forget one has to earn a living. It is also not realised that we have to get up and move at some stage. So as we stand up onto badly positioned feet the problem comes flowing straight back.

Changing exercise routines

Many readers will be athletes, may like to jog or perhaps attend the gym. Pain in the feet be it from *plantar fasciitis* or any of the other myriad of causes can make doing weight-bearing exercises a misery. But with a little willingness we need not lose our fitness which we can maintain in other ways. If you are a regular runner you may like to substitute this for a multi-fitness machine or fast swimming. You may prefer to use a bicycle or a static exercise bike. It is worthy to note that exercise keeps our brains and body in peak condition so we would be wise to avoid abandoning it where possible.

Wobble boards

A wobble board is a fine investment and a great self-help method. It is a rare case that I do not prescribe these at the same time as orthotics to assist greater and quicker recovery. A wobble board will quickly strengthen the muscles in the feet and ankles without danger of overstretch to the plantar aponeurosis, fascia or Achilles. It works by vastly and swiftly strengthening the ankles so that they cease to roll inward into excessive pronation and thus irritate the plantar fascia. You can mimic this effect if you wish to demonstrate pronation on the fascia. To do this push your ankles inward, toward each other, whilst keeping your feet flat on the ground. You will feel a pulling sensation in the arch area. Try to imagine this happening with every step you take! If we can strengthen our ankles we will drastically reduce what is a powerful and destructive irritating factor to the fascia.

The board I choose for patients is fourteen-inches across and the exercises we favour are shown in the following photographs. Remember that during the early days you may care to hold on to something until your balance has improved. We always advocate wearing shoes when doing wobble board exercises.

I recommend three-to-five minutes twice daily for one month, followed by once daily to maintain ankle strength.

Movement 1 "rolling". Keeping the circumference of the board in contact with the ground rotate clockwise, then anti-clockwise.

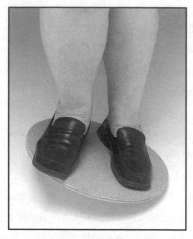

Rolling

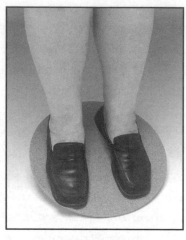

Side to side

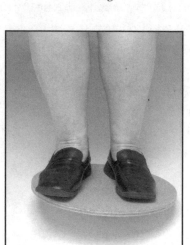

Back to front

Movement 2 "side to side". Literally go side to side, left to right.

Movement 3 "back to front". Rock the board back to front.

Mix all three movements into each session and change from one to the other throughout.

Another exercise – a bit more advanced – is to attempt to balance on the middle peg (but not holding on to anything).

If you wish to make the wobble board a regular thing, it is

well worth paying for a lesson from a physiotherapist or researching the internet where you will find some very interesting variations. To buy a wobble board, again look to the internet or our clinic will happily supply one by mail order (see address at the end of the book). A wobble board is a very worthwhile investment and as well as the uses we advocate them for, they are useful for exercising our balancing skills, as well as our legs and bottom area.

Conclusion

Self-help measures can go toward giving you some relief, and in the case of very acute *plantar fasciitis*, self-help may be all that is needed. You will notice I have purposefully left out off-the-shelf type orthotics. I believe that these merely push the foot from one faulty position to another and have the potential to create pain and even wear and tear in distant areas of the musculoskeletal system. My strong advice is not even to contemplate sending off for, or buying from chemists or the like, any pre made orthotic or arch lift.

CHAPTER EIGHT

OTHER CAUSES OF HEEL PAIN

Not all heel pain is attributable to *plantar fasciitis*, although it has to be said it is rare not to be. Certain types of heel pain can be associated with forms of rheumatoid arthritis, anky-losing spondylitis, and the general rheumatic spectrum of diseases. This goes hand in hand with the rheumatic spec-trums inherent inflammatory nature as well as the general joint laxity that accompanies these diseases. However I will point out that with the correct orthotics I have had astound-ing success with many cases where rheumatic spectrums were an issue. Not all had one hundred per cent success but many were helped fifty to sixty per cent just by skilfully releasing the strain being put on the plantar fascia and Achilles by correcting the individual's gait. Faulty gait coupled with rheumatic spectrum disease processes can lead to joint stress and progressive damage.

There is evidence drawn from some texts that link certain types of heel pain to gout which is caused by a renal excre-tory problem in ninety per cent of cases, or over production of uric acid. The usual site for gout to attack is the hallux (big toe) which presents as hot, red and incredibly tender. In rare cases gout can also affect the subtalar joint, Achilles and heel.

Severs disease is a condition we get to treat in adolescents and its own cause of heel pain is the pulling of the Achilles tendon at its insertion. Although some learned sources say it is caused by minute fractures in the bone at the insertions, it is this author's belief that for all intents and purposes severs disease is merely another form of *plantar fasciitis*, and as such responds in exactly the same way to orthotic treatment.

Retrocalcaneal bursitis occurs as a result of irritation to the bursa sac at the back of the heel. It is usually associated with badly fitting shoes. Generally speaking ultrasound, ice and backless shoes worn for a period of time provide the patient with a satisfactory outcome.

Puncture wounds to the heel may cause infection such as cellulitis, osteomyelitis, osteochrondritis and septic arthritis. A puncture wound can occur where the patient has trodden on a sharp object for example. With infections of this kind, a doctor's advice must be sought.

Direct trauma such as a very high jump or fall onto the heels may give rise to localised fracture at the heel area.

Nerve entrapment of the medial calcaneal nerve elicits pain that travels up the leg and is of a sharp electrical nature. It is thought to be due to excessive pronation of the foot causing micro trauma to the heel.

A dermatome is an area of skin that is fed by a major spinal nerve. Dysfunction of the relevant spinal area will elicit a sensation of numbness and/or pain. The particular dermatome that goes over the heel runs from S1, the first portion of the sacrum. A competent osteopath or chiropractor should be able to carry out relevant tests to determine if a dermatome is the problem.

It must be remembered that the above conditions are relatively rare and even though we as a clinic specialise in heel and foot pain, we seldom ever encounter these conditions.

CHAPTER NINE

OTHER COMMON BIOMECHANICAL FOOT PROBLEMS

I hope you find the following chapter to be useful. I will not go into masses of detail on each condition, but if it stimulates your further reading then I know I will have aroused your interest. Self-diagnosis is never a great idea and a competent practitioner should be sought to confirm, or issue, a valid diagnosis. The recommended reading section at the back of this book will give you a good idea which books to purchase, or borrow from the library, in order to pursue your points of interest further.

There are huge lists of foot conditions we could outline showing many rare and very occasionally seen foot problems, but to keep the interest of the layman I shall seek to give a brief outline of conditions we see and treat on a fairly regular basis.

Metatarsal madness

The most common problem aside from *plantar fasciitis* that I am called upon to treat is metatarsal pain (the ball of the foot). There are a number of metatarsal conditions; the first we shall look at is the dropped metatarsal. Generally the practi-

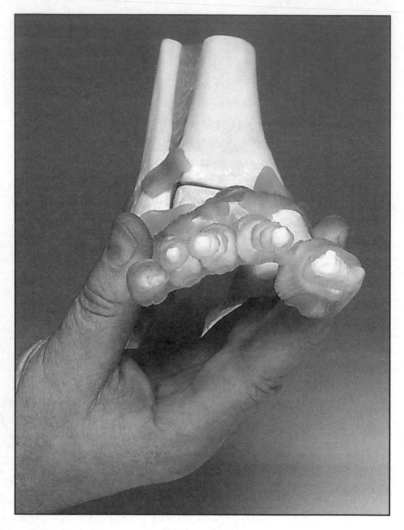

Metatarsal arch

tioner encounters thickened skin over the under surface of the two middle metatarsal heads (the middle section of the ball of the foot). This is where they have been forced downward out of their natural arch (the metatarsal arch). The skin grows into calluses as a protective shell against the ground strike of these two middle metatarsals. This problem is compounded in people who have very little fat layer to the ball of the foot. When we encounter this, the metatarsals are like bony knobs hiding just under the skin. My question as a diagnostician is. Exactly why have these metatarsal heads dropped? Common thought among practitioners is that the ligaments supporting the metatarsal heads merely weaken and allow the dropping effect to occur. I have a major issue with this and always seek to find out why. Generally I will diagnose a problem with the plantar aponeurosis, its surrounding tissues and the unnatural amount of pulling against the metatarsal heads forcing them downward. My own thoughts on this and my clinical findings indicate that metatarsal drop is merely another form of *plantar fasciitis* and indeed in a great majority of cases it accompanies *plantar fasciitis*. It is the normal practice to concentrate on the use of just a metatarsal dome to raise the heads, but my own method is to seek to temper the plantar aponeurosis by correctly balancing the strain upon it and getting it to cease pulling at the metatarsals.

If I had a hammer

We tend to see a lot of hammer toes during our day-to-day practice. These are due to the metatarsal heads being dropped and the unfortunate results are that the toes "claw" to try to stabilise the forefoot in its ground contact. If these are not tackled very early the tendons tend to shorten and even with corrective orthotics the toes need to be straightened either by regular manual manipulation or by surgery in more stubborn examples.

"Me Mortons is killing me Doctor!"

We see hundreds of cases of this vicious little complaint every year. To put it in a nutshell, it's a growth on the nerve or nerves at the point where they run through the metatarsal heads. These will be diagnosed by a practitioner firstly by carrying out a "squeeze test" to the foot which will elicit a sharp pain at the very area the growth is occurring. Secondly ultrasound scanning can be used when there is any doubt. The approach we take is relative to the individual case. For example we are never content to concede that a Morton's neuroma has occurred for no reason in a perfectly biomechanically sound foot. We usually witness pronation causing a "bunching" to the metatarsal heads meaning that the heads squeeze together. It is my belief that the neuroma forms in order to protect the nerve against pressure exerted by the metatarsal heads, one clashing against the other and literally squeezing the nerve. Therefore the approach which seems to yield the best results is first to use an orthotic with a metatarsal dome to raise and space out the heads so as to relieve the burden of pressure on them. Secondly, by correcting pronation and the medial arch we relieve the bunching pressure to the metatarsal heads. Usually this will solve the problem on its own but sometimes the neuroma has got larger and a simple operation is needed to excise it. The orthotic is now needed more than ever as the neuromas will return or further ones will occur without its prudent use. We see many patients with multiple neuromas where operations have been successfully carried out to remove them but the "cause" has not been tackled and further ones have returned.

"Left, right, left right"

The next metatarsal problem is the march fracture which chooses the second/third metatarsal heads as its most frequent site. Of the cases I have dealt with I have found it incredibly rare for the cause not to be associated with dropped metatarsal heads and sometimes including a distinct lack of fat-padding under the metatarsal heads. It is stated in the usual non-enquiring way that it occurs due to over-use in athletes or in soldiers after route marches. I would question this assumption and agree that it happens during these activities but as it does not happen to all soldiers or all athletes then there must be some other intrinsic cause.

"More sugar, Vicar?"

The diabetic foot gives rise to its own problems such as neuropathy (decreased nerve function) or necrosis (circulatory problems associated with blood vessels). People with diabetes mellitus have a naturally increased risk of fracture as bone-mass is reduced. Orthotics as part of the diabetics strict foot health regime must firstly be rigid enough to be effective yet soft enough to avoid the danger of fracture should the person wish to run or do any athletic activity. The softness, particularly in the top cover, is paramount so as not to bruise delicate blood vessels.

The tunnel of love

Tarsal tunnel syndrome is to all intents and purposes carpal tunnel syndrome of the foot (carpal tunnel affects the hand).

It is uncommon and presents with burning pain and numbness in the toes and soles of the foot. Symptoms are usually worst at night. Surgery is a definite indication for this condition and will ensure a rapid recovery.

"I think there's a rod in my toe?"

Hallux rigidus or limitus are conditions in which it is difficult to bend the stiffened big toe. Put simply the joints in the big toe become arthritic; the two joint surfaces wear away leaving osteophytes and semi-fusing the joint. Use of orthotics has been shown to aid hallux rigidus, especially in its infancy, by taking pressure away from the hallux itself. Should this prove to be of only limited use directly, the toe can be fused surgically which generally proves satisfactory. We have usually found a combination of orthotics and physical therapy such as manual traction to the hallux, heat treatment and soft tissue massage to be extremely useful. Shoes worn must be of a kind which will not permit the toe to compact against the end.

"Ooh, me poor ol' bunions!"

Bunions, or more correctly hallux abductor valgus, are either caused by a genetic disposition or a combination of pronation coupled with tight shoes. Genetic factors are thought to account for over half of cases. For example this may be due to an ancestral tendency toward pronation or, as some suggest, the inheritance may be a taste for the wrong type of footwear! The role of orthotics is to take the weight away from the big toe joint and relieve it of pressure. We have found this to be extremely effective clinically, and some reduction in the size of the bunion may even occur. Pain will subside and the bunion will not enlarge further. Surgical intervention will be an option for those who desire the hallux straightened for cosmetic reasons, but this should not be undertaken lightly as, like any surgery, there is a possibility that you may be left in pain. On a more positive note, this procedure is usually very effective and really is a case of personal informed choice.

"Who dares shins!"

Shin splints presents as a pain on the inner (medial) side of the shin bone. It is commonest in runners but can affect anyone with pronation, even those whose only exercise is a walk to the shops for the newspaper. It is a sprain or tear to

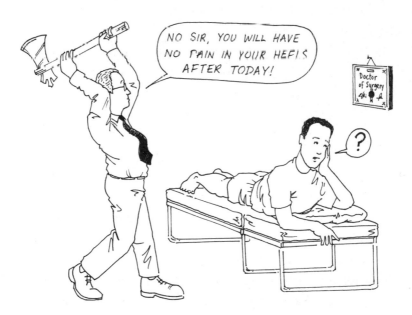

the posterior tibial muscle (8). This originates in the back of your lower leg bone and literally holds your arches up. The cause of true shin splints is that pronation of the foot literally tugs the posterior tibial muscle away from the tibia bone. This progresses and worsens over time. Properly made orthotics are an absolute must and will clear-up shin splint. Accuracy in capturing the non-weight-bearing arch must be strongly emphasised.

It was his weakness . . .

Achilles problems present in many "shapes and sizes" and accurate diagnosis needs to be carried out to assess the type of problem involved. Many Achilles cases where minor injuries are annoyingly frequent should be assessed for biomechanical instability of the foot.

Excessive pronation or rolling at the rear foot may cause a constant strain on an Achilles tendon and pull it into a bow shape when viewed from the rear. This should be assessed and the appropriate orthotic prescribed to straighten the offending "bowing" and release the constant strain.

" 'Anky panky"

The same biomechanical checks we make with Achilles pain must be carried out when there are constant ankle injuries. It will be very likely we have to assess whether pronation would be playing a part by stretching at the ligaments on the inside of the ankle and crushing those on the outer ankle. An orthotic must be used to control this rearfoot pronation and restore the ankle to its comfortable and stable position.

Individual ankle injuries must be assessed by a practitioner for correct diagnosis and treatment, either manually or surgically.

CHAPTER TEN

THE IMPORTANCE OF PROPER ORTHOTICS

As readers have probably gathered, orthotics are a great love of mine having saved me from a lifetime of pain and inactivity due to *Plantar Fasciitis* and shin splints. I thank God every time I run my usual ten miles that I discovered the most incredible orthotics suited one hundred per cent to my indi-

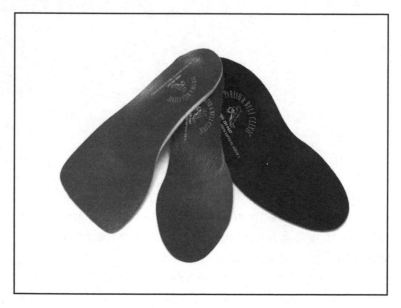

Prescription orthotics

vidual needs, and I remember how I used to suffer sharp pain every time I walked, stood up or hobbled around on waking.

From a practitioner and prescriber point of view, it gives immense pleasure to see patients derive such great benefits from our prescription orthotics, and to receive their thank you letters almost daily still gives me a great thrill and sense of pride. I think all practitioners should feel this, and any doctor or medical person who has lost this should find a new vocation!

One must consider all the alternatives when viewing a patient's condition and should not get tunnel vision that orthotics or indeed any other practice or discipline can be a cure-all. Biomechanical foot problems can only truly be countered by mechanical means, e.g. returning them to a normal stance. Occasionally one requires a wise mixture of surgery or treatment and orthotics to ensure a successful outcome, but in ninety per cent of cases orthotics alone will suffice, perhaps with a little physical therapy.

The term "orthoses" comes from the word "orthos" meaning straight. It is normal thinking amongst most practitioners that a rigid orthotic is the ultimate. I have great argument with this and consider from vast experience of replacing rigid orthotics for patients who have got little or no benefit, or in some instances reacted adversely, that total rigidity in an orthotic is unnecessary. The human foot is designed to move within its limits and even though one corrects the biomechanical fault, it is by design that the orthotic should allow a little movement to remain. It has been shown time and time again that people who live outdoors with bare feet from a young age rarely, if ever, suffer biomechanical foot problems as all the muscles in the feet are going through a constant "workout". My own experience of this first hand was many years ago working with a Thai boxing (or Muay Thai) team. I was osteopath for the team (as well as a fighter at that time) and had the great fortune to be able to observe the feet of this great group of ladies and gents. Bearing in mind that most of these fighters trained for six to eight hours daily in bare feet and all were aged around 18–25, it was interesting to note that their individual foot posture was near perfect.

When we observe traditional Thai boxing training we see that all of it is done balanced on the balls of the feet. So it necessarily follows that all the musculature around the ankles, lower legs and throughout the feet is constantly engaged in pure strength training. In consequence of the above, the feet, with their constant gruelling exercise programme, were able to maintain a perfect posture.

One of those fighters continued as a great friend of mine – long after his active fighting days. It was most interesting to note that within six months of ceasing bare foot training six hours a day his feet had dropped into pronation followed by a pattern of pronatory pains, for which we prescribed orthotics successfully.

The above story illustrates what can be done to strengthen feet from an early age, but for ninety-nine per cent of patients a Muay Thai training school or a Zola Budd running programme is out of the equation!

Many exercises, such as picking up pencils with the toes or rolling the ankles, are given to patients with pronation and dropped medial arches. This approach is akin to carrying out a ten minute gym workout daily and expecting a musculature like that of Arnold Schwarzenegger. The Thai boxing story clearly illustrates the amount of work needed to build foot muscles strong enough to almost "take over" from the lax or overstretched ligaments and support the bodies weight. This would be like expecting to lift a hundred kilos with one bicep muscle.

In view of all this, in a practical normal life we need orthotics to do sixty per cent of the job of the foot's intrinsic strength. To return to the point I was making earlier, the reader will have gathered that the perfect foot has a natural amount of "bounce" or movement and is not to be held solidly, but encouraged to stay "firmly" in its desired position of talar neutral allowing the foot to flex slightly with the orthotic.

At the other end of the spectrum from hard unforgiving orthotic materials, we do not expect major results from a pad-type device. In other words soft orthotics should be discouraged as these prove to be little more than a padding instrument merely adding a squishy layer under the foot. The added problem of these is that they take up a lot of available room in the shoe and limit footwear choice. As a stalwart advocate of correct orthotic devices, I only ever consider these orthotic pads as a temporary measure.

As a clinic, we are constantly appalled at the quality of so-called orthotics which patients who come to us are wearing (these having been prescribed by previous practitioners). Most are rigid, but the models that irritate me the most are the off-the-shelf shells with postings stuck on to emulate a prescription device. The mere fact that the arch bears no resemblance at all to the patients non-weight-bearing foot is immediate evidence of its unsuitability, without the addition of these spurillous paddings and postings that simply cannot add accuracy, as the body of the orthotic is already seriously faulty.

Built on years of observation, my philosophy is that any orthotic that is not specifically designed for your individual foot and all its nuances should never be worn. My reasoning is that one may, if very lucky, adjust the pain of the presenting problem, but the cost to other areas of the muscloskeletal system can be high. I make no apologies for repeating this fact in the book. I want my readers to absorb this thoroughly.

An imperfect foot will cause unnecessary wear and tear and strain to the foot, ankles, knees, hips and lower back. To push the foot from one faulty position to another by using off-the-shelf devices is asking for future problems.

Do not be confused by this text as many "accommodative" devices may be useful; for example, a shielding device for painful bunions or an implement to part the toes and protect against a painful corn. These have a positive place as they do not interfere with Mother Nature's delicate biomechanical balance. At the same time I do like to see, where possible, the causative factor dealt with at the same time as using an accommodative device.

The correct type of orthotic material used is a major factor particularly in dealing with *plantar fasciitis* or problems emanating from the plantar aspect of the foot. Daily, we witness people who consult us with orthotics that put too much pressure to bear against the plantar aponeurosis, which is already inflamed and torn. The orthotic should be able to "give" slightly in its structure particularly under the aponeurosis. With this in mind the orthotic has to support the foot effectively, which means that a mere soft orthotic will be unsuitable.

The ideal orthotic employs a memory shell that will move with the patient's weight and foot type and can be counted on not to lose shape over the years.

When using these materials it is even possible to employ a 1mm gauge material, accurately padded in crucial areas, to give support with inbuilt pertinent flexibility.

A practitioner dealing with orthotics should have a great deal of experience in the use of functional foot orthotics. They should be able to explain fully why an orthotic is needed and be fully conversant with any further options such as surgery or manual treatment. But of utmost importance is the correct knowledge of what steps to take should the orthotic be either painful or not working, for example knowing when to add height to arches (or to lower them), if and when to add or change rear or forefoot support or adjusting paddings etc.

An orthotic laboratory will do most of the work when an orthotic is needed, but it never ceases to amaze us how many practitioners are "lost" when it comes to adjustments. In short, always find a practitioner with a high level of experience and skill.

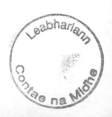

SUMMARY

Each of your feet is a complex tool, capable of great feats of engineering – carrying your frame wherever and whenever you wish to transport yourself somewhere. They slavishly follow instructions from the brain and nervous system, never-ending in their obedience to the user who pushes them thousands of times every day.

When walking, every step carries two-and-a-half times our body weight right through the core of the foot. In the case of a runner one can only guess at the weight ratio per kilo of body weight per foot.

Is it really any wonder that these miracles of nature get biomechanical problems? I have only covered a fraction of the vast list of conditions associated with feet, and then only from a biomechanical point of view. As expressed in the various parts of this book, this is a volume for the layman, but I can thoroughly recommend any of the books I have used as references for your further perusal.

Your feet should receive your every care and attention and when things go wrong only consult the very "cream" of practitioners, use the correct orthotics and if it seems like nothing is helping, keep looking and trying new and better modalities and specialists.

Take the greatest care of yourselves and your feet, and I thank you sincerely for finding the time in your busy life to read my humble volume.

God bless.

Les Bailey
Senior Biomechanics Consultant/Director
Parish and Bell Clinic
46 Banstead Road
Carshalton
Surrey,
SM5 3NW
England

(020) 8395 0447
(020) 8404 6860

www.heelspur.co.uk

REFERENCES

1) Ranowat & Positano, *Disorders of the heel, rearfoot and ankle* (1st edition), Churchill Livingstone, 1999. ISBN 0-443 07838-6.
2) Tontora and Grabowski, *Principles of anatomy and physiology* (9th edition), John Wiley & Sons Inc, 2000. ISBN 0-471-36692-7.
3) *Gray's anatomy* (31st edition), Longmans, 1954.
4) *Dynamic loading of the Plantar Aponeurosis in Walking* Erdemir *et al*, 86 (3) 546.
5) www.arthroscopy.com/sp 09001.htm
6) Dr William Rossi, The arches and some controversial views. www.unshod.org/pfbc/pfrossi.htm
7) *The treatment of 100 common diseases by new acupuncture*, Hong Kong: Medicine & Health Publishing Co, 1988.
8) William Southmayd M.D. and Marshall Hoffman, *Sports health*, Perigee, 1984. ISBN 0-399-51107-5.